Hy... Experience

Insider's Guide to Safe, Healthy and Easier Childbirth

By: Ashley Scott

Author of All Books in **Busy Woman's Natural Birth Series:**

HypnoBirthing - An Introductory Guide
Natural Birth 'Crash Course' - All Women Need to Know, to Feel and Prepare For

HypnoBirthing Experience

Mothers Guide to Safe, Healthy and Easier Childbirth

By: Ashley Scott

Author of Absolute Barbary Womens Natural 30th Session

Alberta, Ardall Canterbury College
Birth, What The Concept Of Womens Need Knowledge of a HypnoBirth

1

Acknowledgement

This Book is dedicated to All Brave Women who took to this Wonderful Path...

Special thanks to those who asked, insisted and assisted me in turning the seminars into this practical form

.

Table of Contents:

"A baby is like the beginning of all things: wonder, hope a dream of possibilities. In a world that is cutting down its trees to build highways, losing its earth to concrete, babies are almost the only remaining link in nature, with the natural world of living things from which we spring."

- Eda J. Leshan

Chapter 1 - Introduction to HypnoBirthing

"Some people come into our lives and quickly go. Some stay for a while, leave footprints on our hearts, and we are never, ever the same." - FlaviaWeedn

HypnoBirthing is not as much a technique as it is a philosophy. HypnoBirthing is not a new concept, but

2

rather a new way to look at the concept of birthing. The philosophy behind HypnoBirthing goes back to Dr. Grantly Dick-Read, who was an English obstetrician in the 1920's. Dr. Dick-Read helped to establish the concept of natural birthing and he was one of the first to move the concept forward.

HypnoBirthing allows you to use the natural birthing muscles just as they were designed to work.

When your body is sufficiently relaxed and you trust in the process, you will be able to allow the process of birth to occur naturally and effortlessly as it was designed to occur.

HypnoBirthing is not a process in which you are in a trance or asleep during the process of birth – it is a process that is akin to daydreaming or focused concentration, similar to what happens when you watch a good movie or become engrossed in a book. If you have ever wondered if HypnoBirthing is for you, then this guide will allow you to make a more informed decision about this most important event in your life. HypnoBirthing allows you to be fully aware and fully in control, because you will be conversant and in good spirits while totally relaxed. HypnoBirthing allows you to feel the surges of birth while surrounded in an atmosphere of calm and relaxation.

This beautiful process helps you alleviate the fear and trauma that can sometimes accompany the process of birth.

As you free yourself from the fear that prevents the muscles of the body from functioning as they were originally designed to function, you allow your body to release those natural endorphins, which are your body's natural relaxant.

Important Facts One Should Know About HypnoBirthing

HypnoBirthing is a childbirth method that helps you prepare for a gentle and comfortable birth.

- It is based on techniques utilized in hypnosis, NLP and guided imagery using positive language and metaphors.

- HypnoBirthing teaches the mother how to release fear and anxiety during labor – utilizing intense relaxation and natural birthing instincts releasing the body's natural endorphins.

- HypnoBirthing can reduce the need for medication and for episiotomy during birth and it can allow the mother to have a shorter labor and birthing.

Common Misunderstanding About Hynobirthing

- One of the greatest fears is that one will not be able to become hypnotized when the moment counts. HypnoBirthing does not mean you are in a deep sleep, during the process as you will be able to speak, to move and to remain in control.

- HypnoBirthing does not require any specific belief system – it is a state of mind that helps you relax and ease away fear and tension.

Hynobirthing Common Questions

How is HypnoBirthing different from other birthing methods?

HypnoBirthing is based on the idea that birthing does not necessarily need to be a painful process. It allows the mother to be properly relaxed and well prepared. Other methods focus more on teaching the mother how to manage and cope with pain. HypnoBirthing allows you to understand that pain is caused by constrictor hormones – these hormones are created by fear - when you learn how to release the fear you then allow your body to release those feel good hormones known as endorphins, natures feel good chemical.

What is a Birth Companion?

A birth companion practices with the mother and helps her prepare for relaxation. The birth companion helps to guide the mother through the process of labor, while helping her with relaxation techniques, visualization and comfort measures amongst other things. The birth companion also helps to welcome the new baby into the world.

Will I be able to comprehend and understand the HypnoBirthing techniques?

HypnoBirthing is a completely natural process – one that you already have access to. The best advice is to approach something like HypnoBirthing with an open mind. Releasing fear is fundamental to the success of the process and the combination of the different methods you will learn like deep breathing, relaxation and visualization, combined with positive thoughts, affirmations and language can help you succeed in just about every area of life – so the effects are long lasting.

How does HypnoBirthing work?

HypnoBirthing allows you to use what is known as the Reticular Activating System, which is a cluster of nerve cells found deep in the brainstem. It has many roles, including the control of essential functions such as breathing and the daily rhythms of the body. The function of the R.A.S. includes its contribution to controlling sleep, walking, sex, eating and elimination. The most important function would be its control of the consciousness and its ability to control sleep, wakefulness, and your ability to focus consciously on things. The R.A.S. serves as a filter by decreasing the possible effects of repeated stimuli like loud noises and it helps prevent overstimulation of the senses, which can help you overcome difficulties.

Will my birth be completely pain free with HypnoBirthing ?

HypnoBirthing is not a guarantee of a pain free birth, however, those that experience the process do find that they have significantly lower levels of pain and this helps them better manage the birthing process.

Fear often contributes to the pain and HypnoBirthing helps you to relax into the process releasing the body's natural endorphins.

Can I still use HypnoBirthing if need medical intervention?

Yes! You will learn some invaluable skills that can help you in many other areas of life beyond child birthing. If you end up needing a medically assisted birth for some reason, you will still find the HypnoBirthing techniques extremely valuable for both you and your baby.

Advantages of HypnoBirthing

You will find there are many advantages to learning about HypnoBirthing . A few of them are listed here:

HypnoBirthing helps:

- Reduce the need for chemical painkillers and other types of drugs.

- Helps alleviate fears by teaching you how to relax deeply.

- Can help shorten the first phase of labor.

- Keep the oxygen flowing to the baby.

- May reduce the need for episiotomy.

- Reduce labor fatigue.

- Helps you embrace the process of pre-birth planning.

- Allows the birth companion to play a significant role.

- Mother and child achieve a gentle, calm and relaxing birth experience.

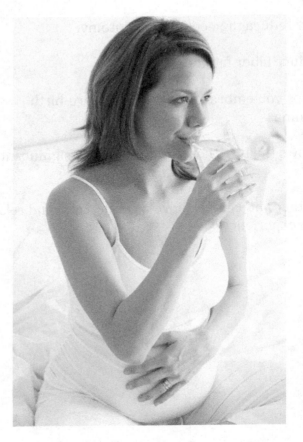

By learning the techniques of HypnoBirthing, you will be able to embrace childbirth instead of fearing it. The techniques learned can help you better understand how your body reacts during childbirth. The process is all about learning how to relax and embrace the birthing process, instead of fearing it.

Chapter 2 – A Short History of Childbirth

"When you change the way you view birth, the way you birth will change." ~Marie Mongan, HypnoBirthing

In our society it is quite difficult to escape the social conditioning that typically surrounds childbirth. Much of the time childbirth is either portrayed as a trauma or a comedy depending on the movies or television shows you watch. What is not portrayed is the experience of how beautiful and natural childbirth can be.

Everywhere a mother turns, she is bombarded by war stories, even from complete strangers as they explain how traumatic their process around birth was.

These types of negative messages can enter your psyche until you really begin to believe that birth is a painful process.

These kinds of stories and pictures can and do become a kind of ingrained belief which causes your mind to keep finding new supporting evidence that shows that the "belief" is true. Our beliefs are at the centre of many of the experiences we have today. Once we believe that childbirth will be a mostly painful experience, then what we believe manifests into our thoughts.

Once we begin to understand the history of childbirth through the ages, and we learn that other cultures don't necessarily have the same attitude towards childbirth that Western society does, we can then begin to see why we our beliefs are not necessarily true.

In Dr.Grantly Dick-Read's 1942 book "Childbirth Without Fear" he states that, "the more civilized the people, the more the pain of labour appears to become intensified". This statement has a lot of relevance when we consider how the non-westernised cultures all over the world birth their babies.

Historically looking at childbirth through the ages, we notice a huge shift in the attitudes and beliefs about birth from before the middle ages compared to after this time. Interestingly enough, it was in the middle ages that Christianity became the dominant religion in Western Society bringing with it massive social change.

Prior to this time in history, birthing was considered one of the highest manifestations of nature – birthing was even considered a rite. It was not considered a painful ordeal it was considered a celebration of life – a celebration in which the community gathered around celebrating the birthing process.

Five Key Points on the Social and Historical Considerations of Childbirth

How Your Ancestors Approached Birth

Our ancestors approached birth much differently than we do. Often times older women or midwives worked with the younger women when they approached birth. Women would most often give birth standing or squatting or even kneeling. Birth was approached and looked at as a natural process.

Midwives who have worked with Aboriginal women are quite surprised at the way in which they labor. More often than not, there are not even any outward signals that these women are about to birth their babies, as the process of birth is a very natural one. In the westernized culture, birth is not typically looked at as such a natural process, but looked at as a complex one.

Women as Healers and Nurturers

Our historical records show that as early as 3000 B.C. that women had their babies quite naturally with a minimum of discomfort with some records showing the entire process taking no more than two to three hours. Up until the time of Aristotle and Hippocrates, women during this time were looked at as healers and nurturers and they often oversaw the role of childbirth.

The Mind-Body Connection and Birth

There is a lot to be said about the mind-body connection and childbirth.

Aristotle even noted the mind-body connection emphasizing the importance of deep relaxation especially during the process of childbirth.

Aristotle and Hippocrates both believed that a woman's feelings, wants and needs during childbirth should be accommodated and they both advocated the importance of women having support during the labor process.

Soranus, another scholar from the Grecian School stressed the importance of women's feelings and needs, similar to Aristotle and Hippocrates. There was typically no mention of pain, except when during an abnormal or complicated birth. Women were treated very kindly and gently during the natural occasion of giving birth and this kind of attitude prevailed for thousands of years.

Birth as a Painful, Lonely and Feared Ordeal

Nearing the end of the second century A.D. there was a widespread wave of contempt against women for some reason even to the point of some misguided people executing midwives, healers and women who had been key to child birthing.

Few avenues were left untraveled as the leaders of the Christian Church set out to redefine the role of women in their society. It was at this time that St. Clement of Alexandria stated: "Every woman should be filled with shame by the thought that she is a woman". The writings, icons or temples that worshipped nature were also destroyed along with the concept that childbirth was a natural process.

Since that time, it became law that women, who were once reveled and supported, were now segregated during pregnancy and isolated for childbirth. Some were labeled as seductresses and pregnancy was seen as the product of "carnal sin".

Birth, which was once celebrated and welcomed, had eroded into a very painful, lonely and much to be feared ordeal, and this was to remain the norm for hundreds of years.

In the sixteenth century, Martin Luther wrote, "If women become tired, or even die, it does not matter. Let them die in childbirth. That's what they are there for." This is obviously quite a shift in attitude towards women and the process of birthing!

Fear and Impact on Labor and Childbirth

All of these events are key to understanding how our fears have developed over time as it pertains to childbirth. Childbirth, once reveled and celebrated became something that was now feared. Fear creates tension, which then creates labor complications.

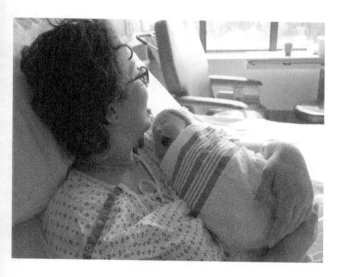

This fear has continued to infiltrate generations of women and it continues to play out strongly in our society today. It also continues to negatively impact labor and more often than not, unnecessarily.

Chapter 3 – How Hypnosis Plays a Role in Birth

"When you have come to the edge of all light that you know and are about to drop off into the darkness of the unknown, FAITH is knowing one of two things will happen: There will be something solid to stand on or you will be taught to fly" ~Patrick Overton

What is Hypnosis?

Hypnosis is a misunderstood state of mind. Many people shy away from it because they lack an understanding of it. Alternative therapies like hypnosis are becoming much more accepted. The truth of the matter is that all hypnosis is essentially self-hypnosis because one must allow oneself to be hypnotized.

Hypnosis is a process that uses the mind-body-connection to influence the subconscious mind.

It is an essentially an altered state of consciousness in which one has an increased intensity of awareness. Hypnosis has also been defined as focused concentration.

19

When you allow a practitioner to 'hypnotize' you, that is hypnosis. When you develop the techniques and learn how to bring your own mind into that same state of focused relaxation, you are also experiencing hypnosis, the only difference is that it is self induced.

Many people use hypnosis to bring about a state of calm and to promote healing. Guided Imagery, which is also a form of trance, is used all of the time in the health care system to help patients visualize themselves healing, and this process is similar to hypnosis. Other similar states of mind include visualization, meditation and even NLP, neuro-linguistic programming.

In the end, the only person that can 'hypnotize' you is YOU and that's an important fact to keep in mind. You are always in control with hypnosis and HypnoBirthing .

Each of us goes in and out of different states of trance on a regular basis every time we miss an exit on the highway or get lost in thought. Anything that causes our mind to wander stimulates our imagination creating a suggestible state; all of which could be classified as a form of hypnosis.

States of Consciousness - Brainwave States

Hypnosis has been around for hundreds of years dating as far back as Ancient Egypt.

The conscious and unconscious, or subconscious mind, are two very different things. Hypnosis is an absolutely incredible and amazing way to make changes in your life and it is a very simple process. Hypnosis changes your thinking and your thought process at a very deep level of the mind, allowing you to easily and effortlessly make changes

Sigmund Freud, although he certainly did not invent the idea of the conscious versus the unconscious mind, did make it very popular and better known. Freud compared the mind to an iceberg in the fact that the conscious mind only represents the very tip of the iceberg. The unconscious mind or that which lies below our conscious thoughts stores a much vaster amount of information. He believed that while we are fully aware of what is going on in the conscious mind, most of us have little to no idea of what kind of information is stored in the unconscious mind.

Our minds actually go in and out of different brainwave frequencies on a regular basis.

The Alpha brainwave state is the state most often accessed during trance or deep relaxation. The Beta brainwave state is the primary state of mind most of us are in during the course of our day and the Beta brainwave state typically resonates around 12 to 40 Hz.

The Alpha brainwave state corresponds to a frequency level around 8 to 12 Hz, which is slower than the Beta state. The Alpha brainwave state is often associated with an extremely relaxed state of mind and this relaxed state of mind is very conducive to suggestion.

The Theta brainwave state is even slower than Alpha and it occurs around 4 to 8 Hz. Theta is a very deep state of relaxation and even light sleep and it is the state of mind most often accessed during meditation and deep levels of hypnosis.

One of the deepest and slowest brainwave states is Delta and it occurs around 0 to 4HZ. Delta brainwave states usually arise in very deep sleep, and this level of mind is not typically accessed during hypnosis.

Hypnosis versus Relaxation and Meditation

According to Albert Einstein, imagination is even more important than knowledge.

The subconscious mind does not know the difference between imagination and reality, so when you replay a scenario in your mind, the mind takes it as fact. Hypnosis is very similar to relaxation and meditation. Unlike meditation or simple relaxation, hypnosis allows you to focus on a certain goal you may have in mind. You might even call it a supercharged form of meditation.

Visualization and self-hypnosis are very powerful tools and you can literally use them to change your life. When you can learn to use your imagination you begin to convert thoughts and feelings into mental images. Those mental images are perceived as reality by the subconscious mind, so eventually the mind brings those mental images into your world.

When you begin to see things in your mind's eye you bring those things into your reality. When you can feel it, see it, taste it and experience it in your mind, you send a powerful signal out to the world through your energy. Our thoughts really do become things - there is simply a time delay in which they manifest.

Hypnosis can help you use the incredible power of your mind to help you relax into the process

of labor. It helps create a sense of calm helping you stay focused.

Hypnosis can help you work with the rhythm of your body so that you can work with the surges of birth rather than against them.

Using a tool like HypnoBirthing allows you to reduce or modify your perception of pain, helping diminish your fears and anxiety. HypnoBirthing can also help you learn how to focus and relax during the birthing process, reducing the need for medical intervention. Hypnosis works by helping the mother expand her emotional and mental control in labor, smoothing the transition and helping to welcome the baby into the world.

The birth of a child is much more than a mere physical process. Birth has both personal and social significance for both the mother and the birth partner and their roles and relationships are forever altered as a result of the birth experience. The goal of a tool like HypnoBirthing is to support the natural physical process of birth, helping to provide a meaningful experience for both the mother and the birth partner.

Birth does not need to be something you fear, it should be something you welcome.

Using a tool like HypnoBirthing ,you are able to tap into the zone as your fears and anxieties associated with childbirth are released. Fear creates tension and tension can in turn cause a taut cervix – and a taut cervix cannot perform its natural function. When the mother is relaxed and calm, her cervix is relaxed and calm as well, allowing the natural process of birth to move forth.

Chapter 4 - The Affect of Fear on Birth

"My baby is healthy and innately knows when to begin labor. My body knows how to birth by instinct. My mind has released all fears and trusts birth. I am enjoying this process and growing through it all." ~Mrs. BWF

The Fight or Flight Stress Response

The stress response, otherwise known as the fight or flight response plays an integral role in something like childbirth.

When you feel fear, your body automatically activates certain hormones including adrenaline, cortisol and others; this in turn releases glucose into the blood stream for energy as needed. When you feel fear in the body, this creates muscular tension amongst other types of issues. When you are relaxed and calm and in the zone, your muscles are more relaxed also.

Any type of fear, whether it is perceived or real can trigger or cause the stress response. Getting into the zone with hypnosis triggers the relaxation response, which moves the body from a state of physiological arousal to a state of peace and calm where the blood pressure decreases, the heart rate slows and the breathing becomes slower and much more relaxed.

It is absolutely impossible to feel stressed and relaxed at the same time.

Stress and anxiety are something we all have to deal with on a day-to-day basis. We usually only become aware of something like stress when it begins to overwhelm us in some way. When we sense danger, whether it is real or imagined, our body's fight or flight response and our nervous system kicks into high gear.

Our bodies are well equipped to handle most types of stressful situations but too much stress can cause us to break down.

In a sense, stress is our body's warning system and it is a signal that something needs to be addressed. Short bursts of stress can actually strengthen our immune system and stress can also help us with our motivation levels by kicking us into high gear helping us get things done.

But, too much stress can be a very bad thing. Stress releases special hormones in the body, called cortisol, which can create all kinds of issues from tension in the body, fatigue, weight gain, fogginess, sleepless nights, and so much more.

Turning on the relaxation response using hypnosis as a tool is a wonderful way to get the mind and body in sync helping one enjoy the process of giving birth.

Getting into the Zone While Birthing

Using hypnosis, one can easily get into the zone while birthing. Woman have been giving birth for hundreds of years in a very natural and normal way. Our bodies can adjust to this process naturally by allowing us to go into the zone. By focusing intently on the process of birth we can tap into that inborn power within.

"Childbirth brings a change in the state of consciousness akin... to that achieved by shamans and mystics. It is a time when a woman reaches beyond normal perceptions and may involve a vision of the universe which transcends ordinary reality."

From Birth Traditions & Modern Pregnancy, by Jacqueline Vincent-Priya

Certain medical technologies and interventions have lessoned our natural instincts and our strengths when it comes pregnancy and birth.

Utilizing hypnosis allows you to easily and effortlessly tap into that state of mind that allows you to focus on what is important, the act of giving birth in a natural and beautiful way.

Sympathetic Nervous System

In order to further understand how hypnosis works, we must first understand how the nervous system works.

There are two distinct nervous systems in the human body– the Central Nervous System and the Autonomic Nervous System. The Central Nervous System or CNS is the processing center of the nervous system - it utilizes the brain and the spinal cord.

The Autonomic Nervous System or ANS regulates the functions of your internal organs such as the heart, the stomach and the intensities. The ANS has two divisions, the sympathetic and the parasympathetic nervous system.

The sympathetic nervous system or SNS controls your ability to respond to emergencies – in other words it is your fight or flight syndrome. The SNS controls your heart rate, your respiration and even your blood pressure. This system also releases adrenaline to give you energy if you need it during an emergency. The SNS can also come into play when you are nervous or anxious.

Parasympathetic Nervous System

The parasympathetic nervous system or PNS creates the opposite response. It slows down the rate of the heart, the blood pressure and even the respiration. The PNS restores the body to a state of peace of calm so that the body can conserve energy.

These two systems cannot operate at the same time therefore utilizing hypnosis you can activate the PNS in order to help your mind and body to relax. When you are able to relax deeply, you are able to tap into the subconscious mind, where changes are more easily made. Using your imagination, you can envision yourself going through the birthing process with ease.

Keeping fear at bay is integral to the process of birth.

When you are stressed or afraid for some reason, you tend to secrete hormones that delay or even inhibit the process of birth. Knowledge is power, so arming yourself with knowledge as it pertains to the process of giving birth can go a long way to helping you enjoy the process for what it is – a miracle.

Even your past fears can get in the way and keep you from enjoying the process. As we have seen, fear creates the fight or flight response which can impact the overall experience of birth.

Fear creates:

- The fight or flight response.

- Tension, anxiety and pain.

- Postpartum it can create confusion, a feeling of helplessness and even anxiety.

In life fear is an obstacle to your happiness and your ability to create and thus enjoy success.

Even if you have previously experienced a fear filled birth, it doesn't mean that your next one will be the same.

With hypnosis, you can delve into your feelings and discover why you react the way you react.

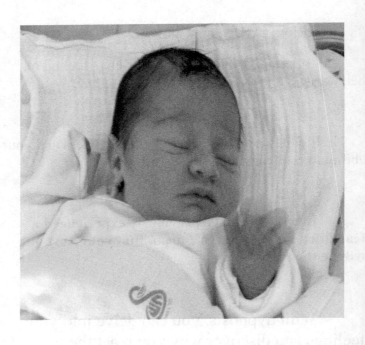

Using the power of your memory, you can change the way you think and feel about the birth experience. By working with and modifying those memories, you can break through those barriers that are keeping you from enjoying the beautiful experience of giving birth.

Chapter 5 – Labor Progression Facts You Need to Know

"There is a secret in our culture, and it's not that birth is painful. It's that women are strong." ~ Laura Stavoe Harm

The Stages of Labor

Each stage of the labor process brings with it new experiences.

This is an important time for the practitioner as well as the birth partners. As each stage of labor progresses it is important for the mother to be fully equipped and supported. The job of the practitioner and/or birth partner is to teach them how and when to apply the skills they have learned.

The initial stage of labor typically begins at home – it may also be referred to as early labor. As the surges begin, progress becomes stronger and more frequent. There are many ways to help the birth mother cope effectively within these surges.

For every surge, a technique known as "surge breathing" has been shown to be very effective.

Another technique used frequently is known as the "balance breath" – and it can also be very effective for centering the birth mother.

Having a written list of positive affirmations or statements, which we will talk about a little bit later, is also an important part of the process. These positive statements are simply statements that represent the state of mind that the mother wants to be in at the present time. Light touch massage may be intermittently used as well, whenever the birth mother desires.

The first stage of labor includes the thinning out or effacement of the cervix to 10 cm.

This stage includes the latent phase and the active phase. The latent phase of labor, known as pre-labor, involves the thinning out of the cervix to 4 cm. It is usually characterized by mild surges and lower back discomfort.

The surges during this period are generally short lasting about 10-20 seconds – they can be mild and irregular as well. Each experience will be unique, as the pattern of surges stop and start, affecting the length of the labor itself. For first time mothers the cervix needs to efface or thin prior to the dilation. For mothers that have been through the birth process before, the thinning and dilation will happen simultaneously. This stage is also referred to as pre-labor.

The second stage of labor will typically involve going to the hospital, unless of course the mother is choosing a home birth.

As the surges grow more frequent, and the uterus continues to soften, the cervix opens allowing for the smooth transition of the baby.

When the cervix is fully dilated and it reaches 10 cm the next stage of labor begins. The second stage of labor occurs when the cervix is fully dilated. Everyone experiences each stage of labor very differently, so these stages are merely a guide.

Each uterine surge begins at the top of the uterus and spreads across and down the organ, which is very muscular. The mother may feel these surges low and in the front of her abdomen and they may also spread through the vagina and lower back.

This cycle repeats itself allowing the birth mother to rest between surges. The period of rest will vary, as the mother gets closer to the next stage of birth. As the labor progresses, the rest periods will vary from 20-30 minutes to a mere 1-minute during the active phase of labor.

Labor is a continuous process characterized by the surge and retraction of the uterus causing the muscle cells to become shorter, which in turn makes the uterus smaller in order to push the baby down and out.

With each surge, the uterus tilts forward and down while the cervix simultaneously thins and opens gradually.

The process of labor is a pattern that will differ with each mother.

The active phase of labor causes the cervix to dilate more rapidly. The surges then become stronger and more rhythmic. The transition phase begins when the cervix reaches 8-10 cm. This next stage is also known as the pushing stage. Surges become very intense at this stage as well. At this point the mother's water will most likely break, causing a warm gush of fluid to be expelled. The mother may also experience what is known as the bloody show, which is the secretion of the mucus plug.

As the baby moves down the birth canal, the baby rocks back and forth which allows adequate time for the pelvic floor muscles and the perineum to gradually stretch. When the baby's head and shoulders emerge from the birth canal, it is called crowning.

The active phase of labor may take 1-2 hours for new mothers, but it may be much faster for those who have already given birth. The third stage of labor occurs as soon as the baby is delivered.

At this point, the placenta and membranes are delivered, this is also known as afterbirth. Depending on your level of care, this stage of birth may be actively managed or allowed to occur naturally.

Hormones and Labor

After the delivery of the baby the birth mother has a natural surge of oxytocin, a hormone, as she and baby begin the bonding process. Allowing for skin-to-skin contact helps promote this release of hormones.

This surge also helps the uterus contract helping to release the placenta from the wall of the uterus. The umbilical cord is left intact until the cord stops pulsating. Once the placenta is fully separated from the uterine wall, both the membranes and the placenta are pushed downward and are delivered via a final urge to push.

The most important thing to remember is that this process is different for each and every birth mother, and the style of management must meet the needs of the birth mother.

The Uterus and Labor

The bones and muscles of the pelvis help support the growing baby/uterus. The uterus surrounds the baby and both the uterus and the baby grow simultaneously. The cervix is a part of the uterus but made up of much different tissue. As the mother approaches birth, the cervix, which is normally thick and closed during pregnancy, becomes thinner – this is also known as effacement.

The vagina leads from the cervix to the outside of the woman's body, allowing for the baby to pass through.

There are 3 muscular layers of the uterus and each of these layers works together to help birth the baby.

The outer layer is known as the Perimetrium, and it consists of longitudinal, smooth thick muscle fibers that work in a strong wave-like pattern. This pattern is more prominent in the upper portion of the uterus. The function of these muscle fibers is to contract and retract - drawing up the lower portion of the uterus and moving the baby down the birth canal.

The middle muscular layer is called the Myometrium and it consists of circular muscle fibers found mainly in the lower portion of the uterus/cervix. These fibers are longer and thinner allowing the longitudinal fibers to stretch and the cervix to progressively open, merging at the lower segment of the uterus. The pressure created by the baby's head also helps this process.

The various birth hormones work to help soften the ligaments that are between the bones in the pelvis.

During this time the mother may feel sore and achy and she may even feel a shift in her balance.

The stages of labor:

First stage involves dilation – surges work to open the cervix up.

2nd stage involves pushing, surges work to bring the baby into the birth canal and vagina.

Third stage involves delivering the placenta and after birth.

Things that can influence the progression of the labor process, the four P's of labor:

The **"Passenger,"** the baby.

The **"Passage,"** the bones of the pelvis, muscles in the pelvis and the cervix and vagina.

The **"Power"** of surges.

The **"Psyche,"** your emotional state of mind.

Chapter 6 – The Power of Breathing

"If you want to conquer the anxiety of life, live in the moment, live in the breath." — Amit Ray, Om Chanting and Meditation

Everything in our lives begins with breathing. Breathing is the foundation and basis for everything we will do during the course of our lives. Without our breath, we cannot survive and we certainly cannot thrive.

The breath is our elixir of life.

There are a few things we can live without, however, breathing is obviously not one of them. Breathing is one of those things we often take for granted. If all of a sudden, we could not breathe, it would not be long before the mere act of breathing became our number one priority.

When you think about it, breathing is one of the most powerful resources you can tap into. It is the basis of all life. Every living thing on the planet breathes. Breathing is one of those few functions of the body, which is controlled at both the conscious and unconscious levels of the mind.

The Many Benefits of Breathing:

Breathing releases stress and tension.

Breathing helps us detoxify the body.

Breathing relaxes our mind, body and spirit.

Breathing gives us more life force energy, also known as chi.

Proper breathing increases our oxygenation and our blood circulation.

Breathing can help us release emotional problems and destructive patterns.

Breathing brings us about a state of peace and euphoria.

Breathing can help us release our physical pain and accelerate healing.

Now let's examine some of the different types of breathing techniques associated with HypnoBirthing.

The Balance Breath

The balance breath helps one feel centered and balanced. It can be used between surges or anytime one would like to feel more grounded. The goal of the balance breath is to achieve half the inhalation to the exhalation.

To practice the balance breath, one would simply breathe in to a count of four and slowly breathe back out to a count of eight. The balance breath helps one achieve the alpha brainwave frequency, which is a slower and much more relaxing state of mind than our normal waking state.

Some Guidelines for the Balance Breath

- Place fingertips so they meet gently at the top of the abdomen – this can help direct the breath.
- Don't rush – perform the breathing pattern slowly and rhythmically.
- The balance breath is best done inhaling though the nose.
- Exhale through the nose or mouth.
- May feel sleepy after 4-5 breaths.

The Surge Breath

The surge breath is a very important breath for labor as well. The surge breath is equal amounts of inhalation to exhalation. The goal of the surge breath is to achieve 3 - 4 breaths in 60 seconds. The surge breath can be utilized with each surge.

The surge breath helps increase oxygen to the body, which in turn helps oxygenate the baby. This important breath also helps reverse the fight or flight stress response.

Some Guidelines for the Surge Breath

One can perform one long inhalation and one long exhalation.
Can count from 1 –10 during both inhale and exhale.
Don't worry about not doing it correctly - just get into the flow.The numbers are merely a guide.
The surge breath is best done inhaling through the nose. Exhalation can occur through the nose or mouth.

One can also practice a little visualization during the surge breath by imagining the breath traveling down into the body.

This can be done by imagining the breath as a beautiful color, filling up the lungs and then crossing the placenta into the baby's system vitalizing the baby. Upon exhalation, visualize a different color.

The Birth Breath

The birth breath is a very important breath for the 2nd stage of labor. It is a deeper and fuller inhalation that is done much more slowly than the surge breath or the balance breath. The goal of the birth breath is to use it with the momentum and the energy of the surge – this helps to increase oxygen to the woman's body while also helping the baby. It helps a woman to increase efficacy of the surge also because it helps her work with her body's natural momentum.

Some Guidelines for the Birth Breath

- One can perform a deep inhalation and a longer, slower exhalation.
- Try imagining a coffee press or plunger in the belly. Upon exhaling, see the plunger being pressed down into the body with the energy of the breath.
- Imagine the breath as it travels down into the body, filling the lungs.
- Try to keep the breath flowing.

The birth breath is best done inhaling through the nose. Exhale through the nose or mouth.

It is clear that the act of breathing can help the mother regain control during the birthing process. Breathing can help detoxify the body giving the mother much needed energy.

We consciously control our breathing when we engage in activities like meditation, yoga or speech. At the unconscious level, our breathing is automatically regulated by certain centers in our brainstem.

Breathing can help us relax and gain control in times of stress and it is certainly an integral part of the birthing process.

Chapter 7 – The Effect of Language on Birthing

Life is not measured by the number of breaths we take, but by the moments that take our breath away. – Origin Unknown

Specific HypnoBirthing Language

The language we use is an important part of the birth experience.

Words and language play an integral role in our lives and they also play a critical role in the birthing process.

Our language impacts everything we do and it also affects our feelings. The language we use allows us to interact with other people and it gives us the ability to express ourselves.

Each and every culture has a different subset of language. In order to understand one another, we must communicate via language. Communication can be verbal or non-verbal, and the way in which we communicate says a lot about our feelings. Our brains process information based on what we hear as well as the emotions that are attached to the words.

In HypnoBirthing , there is an important relationship between the birthing process and language.

HypnoBirthing uses what is called non-threatening words. These kinds of words allow the mother to experience much less anxiety and fear as it pertains to the birthing experience. As we have seen, the birth experience can be very traumatic if we allow it to.

Positive language and words helps us decondition the mind and it helps us focus on the positive and beautiful aspects of birth, rather than the negative.

Positive language and words utilized in HypnoBirthing

- Surge or wave versus contraction.
- Pressure/sensation or tightening versus pain.
- Birth companion versus coach.

- Membranes Release versus Water Breaking/Rupturing.
- Energy breath versus pushing.
- Unborn baby versus fetus.
- Parents versus patient.
- Newborn versus neonate.
- Birthing month versus due date.
- Special circumstances versus complications.
- Birthing versus labor.
- Uterine Seal versus mucous plug.
- Thinning/Opening versus Effacing or Dilating.
- Birth versus deliver.
- Pre-Labor Warm-Up versus Braxton Hicks
- Pelvic Floor Exercises versus Kegals.

These types of words help alleviate fear and anxiety.

Utilizing non-medical words versus medical words can go a long way to helping the mother focus on the positive. These types of words also help reprogram the mind and the brain arming the mother with the tools required for relaxation and comfort.

Language plays an important role in this process, as you can see. Since the mind can only hold onto one image or thought at a time, opposing thoughts are blocked out if one is focused on the positive. That being said, when you focus on positive and affirming thoughts, you change the energy in and around you, creating a more positive mindset.

Since our thoughts precede our reality, whatever we focus on comes into being.

The thoughts we think are in a sense imprinted onto our subconscious mind, helping us move through the experiences in life in a much more positive manner.

The Role of Self-Hypnosis

You might be wondering how a tool such as self-hypnosis plays into HypnoBirthing. Self-hypnosis can help the birth mother relax and better experience the process of giving birth. The state of relaxation that is achieved during self-hypnosis will change the way the birth mother experiences the birth process.

Self-hypnosis is very easy to learn and it can go a long way to helping the mother reduce fear and alleviate pain. Hypnosis is a tool that can help one achieve a state of deep relaxation. The goal of self-hypnosis in a process such as HypnoBirthing is to empower the mother to allow for a more relaxing birth experience.

Hypnosis helps reduce stress and it also helps alleviate the negative connotation often associated with the birthing process. Self-hypnosis allows the body to relax allowing the subconscious mind to work at its full potential, distracting the mind from any negative thoughts and feelings.

Affirmations can also be utilized in this process as well. Positive affirmations, as we learned before, are simple statements set in the present tense and they reflect the state of mind one wishes to be in or achieve.

Some common affirmations that can be used in HypnoBirthing are:

• I relax my mind and body so that I can easily birth my baby.

• My mind and body work together in complete harmony.

• I trust that my body knows exactly how to birth my baby.

• I am focused on a calm and smooth birth.

As long as the statements are written from a positive perspective, the subconscious mind can accept it. Positive affirmations can be written or spoken, and they are typically prepared prior to beginning self-hypnosis.

The more we focus on positive thoughts and images, the more those images become a part of our subconscious mind, changing the world around us.

Chapter 8 – VAK Techniques

We are what we repeatedly do. Excellence, then, is not an act, but a habit. – Aristotle

VAK – Visual, Auditory and Kinesthetic Techniques

Our minds process things differently depending on whether or not we sense things in a visual, auditory or kinesthetic manner.

This is also what is known as VAK. Each of us sees things from a different perspective.

If for example, you are an auditory person you most likely use your sense of hearing rather than your sense of sight. In other words, you may relax more while listening to soothing music as opposed to thinking of a picture or a scene like a beach. If you process information in a visual manner, you probably love the idea of a beautiful serene beach, because you can actually see the beach in your mind's eye. If you are more of a kinesthetic processor, or one who processes information via touch or feel, you might like to imagine yourself touching the sand or imagine yourself walking with your feet immersed in the water.

We all have unique filters through which we see the world depending on the experiences we have had in our lives.

Most of us tend to think in one particular mode over another: visual, auditory or kinesthetic. There are actually two additional modes, but they are not as common - olfactory and gustatory.

If you tend to see images in your mind when someone asks you a question, you more than likely prefer the visual mode. If you respond better to sounds and words, you probably prefer the auditory response mode. If you love the touch and feel of a beautiful piece of fabric you probably lean towards the kinesthetic mode. The kinesthetic processor is also more likely to feel emotions rather than hearing or seeing something. These three modalities are also described as site, sound and touch. Olfactory senses have to do with our sense of smell while gustatory receptors have to do with our sense of taste.

Think about how you remember people for a moment? Do you recall how sultry someone's voice is? Perhaps you are an auditory processor. Maybe you see someone's face and recall how handsome or beautiful they are, that may mean you are a visual processor. If you recall the sense of touch more, you would most likely remember how wonderful someone feels as you imagine a warm embrace.

Each of these modalities can be utilized in HypnoBirthing. Once you understand how someone sees the world, you can then change your speech and your behaviors to match theirs. Let's look at some of the techniques now and how they play into HypnoBirthing .

Visual Techniques – The Power of Visualization

What exactly is Visualization? In simple terms it is just a mental image that is similar to a visual perception. It is a very powerful tool that has been used for hundreds of years to promote relaxation and to reduce and eliminate pain. Visualization techniques can be a very powerful healing mechanism. When we think and visualize ourselves accomplishing something, like giving birth in a positive and healthy manner for example, we are much more likely to move into that state of mind.

Our brains create thoughts, words and images that can then be used in conjunction with our imagination.

This makes thoughts and images extremely powerful. Our brain can create any image that we can imagine. During hypnosis these powerful images can greatly affect our subconscious mind helping us achieve any goal.

It is important to note that the mind and body respond to whatever image it is presented with, whether or not that image is real or imagined. During labor and childbirth, these kinds of tools can be extremely helpful. During labor, for example, a woman can visualize herself having a positive birth experience.

Typical Visualization Tools

- Visualize the muscles and layers of the uterus working together.

- See the outer layer gently drawing up and pushing the baby down.

- See the inner layer gently releasing and relaxing.

- Visualize that oxytocin flowing.

- See oxygen coming into the body, flowing to your baby.

- See the baby gently floating, waiting to meet you.

- Visualize yourself somewhere peaceful like a garden or natural pool of water.

Auditory Techniques - The Power of Affirmations

Auditory techniques are also important when it comes to birthing your baby. Auditory techniques like affirmations can be repeated silently or spoken out loud. As we have seen, affirmations are statements that affirm what we want to be true or what we believe to be true. They are always stated in a positive manner in the present tense, as if they have already occurred.

Affirmations can be a very valuable tool when it comes to adding another layer of positivity to the birthing process.

Affirmations can be useful during pregnancy, during the pre labor process and also after the baby is born. Affirmations can help condition the mother so she is set up for success. During the labor process, audio tracks can be used combined with affirmations to help the mother block out intrusive sounds of the hospital environment. Affirmations are a positive influence on the brain chemistry and they are very simple to create and use. Affirmations should only be used and repeated by the birth partner during the active phase of labor if the mother specifically requests it – otherwise they could prove to be distracting.

Typical Affirmations

- I trust my body, and I follow its lead.
- I am relaxed and happy that my baby is coming to me.
- I am focused on a smooth and calm birth.
- My mind and body are relaxed.
- I feel confident, safe and secure.
- I now turn my birthing over to my body and my baby.
- I breathe deeply and fully.
- I welcome my baby with great happiness and joy.
- I focus on what I can do then I do it.
- I relax my mind and my body so that I can birth my baby.
- My baby is at ease because I am at ease.
- My body and baby work together in harmony.
- My body is perfectly designed to give birth and it does so well.
- I feel the sensations of labor and know that everything is fine.
- I love my baby and I'm doing all I can to prepare for a healthy, smooth birth.
- I trust my body knows exactly how to birth.
- I feel calm and relaxed.

Kinesthetic Techniques

Kinesthetic techniques can also be used during the labor and delivery process. They can be very soothing for the mother as well. Touching and feeling techniques are a great way to help the mother feel connected while she is birthing her baby.

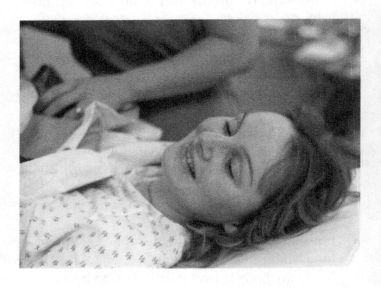

Kinesthetic techniques help condition the mother and they also serve as a positive influence on the body chemistry, helping to release endorphins and enable relaxation. These kinds of techniques can also be used to help the mother sleep in the months prior to labor and delivery.

Types of Kinesthetic Techniques

Surge Techniques – The surge technique is designed to be used while the mother is in labor. Once again, this technique should only be used if the mother requests it.

Place the hand on the mother's forehead with a steady but gentle pressure – slowly stroke the forehead. Perform a light arm touch from the wrist to the shoulder, doing a slow touch up the arm and back down again.

Gently press the shoulder or shoulders when the mother exhales.

Light Touch Massage – used mainly on the back during surges or during longer periods of time.

Helps the body release endorphins acting as an analgesic.

Very relaxing.

Works on the Gate Theory – The Gate Theory, which was proposed in the 1960's, proclaimed that the spinal cord contains a neurological "gate" that controls pain signals. This so called "gate" either blocks signals or sends the signals through.

There are two kinds of light touch massage, the Criss Cross or Figure Eight and the V's. These kinds of techniques help the body release endorphins, which can be just as powerful as painkillers like morphine. Endorphins can also help relieve stress, ease away depression and boost self-esteem.

Chapter 9 – The Role of The Birth Partner

"The knowledge about how to give birth is born within every woman: women do not need to be taught how to give birth but rather to have more trust and faith in their own body knowledge." – BirthWorks

Helping Your Partner Relax

There are many advantages to having a birth partner. The birth partner plays a significant role in the birth process. **The birth partner or companion helps the mother gently welcome the baby into the world, providing invaluable support.**

The birth partner's role is to support the mother throughout the entire process of labor and delivery so they must be familiar with all parts of the birthing process from relaxation and breathing to the final moments of delivery. Their role is to provide care and compassion, be of assistance or to simply hold the mother's hand providing reassurance. They also help the mother and offer emotional support during labor, help with various breathing techniques, assist in providing comfort and reassurance while helping to facilitate communication between the mother and the care providers. It is important for the birth partner to nurture and protect the mother's memory of the birth experience as well.

As the mother's labor progresses, the birth partner helps to calm and reassure the mother that everything is progressing smoothly.

The birth partner may also help in the creation of a birth rehearsal, which may involve deciding on birth techniques, choosing pain relief methods if any and offering emotional support. The birth partner's presence helps to decrease anxiety and encourage the mother.

The birth partner is essentially the guardian of the birthing room, acting as a liaison between the mother and the delivery or the hospital staff.

The birth partner acts a coach and a partner, helping to reinforce the learning and techniques that help ensure a smooth delivery.

Light Touch Massage Techniques

The light touch massage is very relaxing, but as we have seen, it also helps stimulate the production of the body's feel good pain relieving chemicals known as endorphins. A good way to gauge when this occurs is the response that the body feels when someone lightly touches or massages the back - creating what is more commonly known as goose pimples. This is a good sign that the body is releasing those incredible endorphins.

Light touch massage is done to the skin and it can be done directly on the skin or through a thin layer of clothing – much of this depends on the mother's preference. Light touch massage can be done during labor surges or any other time the mother so desires.

The best way to do a light touch massage is in a rhythmical manner and pattern remaining consistent with the touch. One important thing to remember is not to constantly stop and start because consistency is the key to a good massage. Those who usually prefer deep tissue massage will also enjoy this technique.

There are basically two approaches to the light touch massage. Both of these approaches involve the birth partner standing behind the birth mother using the back of the fingertips creating a light and consistent rhythmic pressure.

The relaxation massage or light touch massage focuses on releasing tension through soft and very gentle repetitive strokes. The technique combines both ancient eastern and western techniques and it is based on the idea that the touch is very therapeutic. By allowing the body to release endorphins it helps to lessen the pain perception while also producing a general relaxation and euphoria.

There are two ways one can perform a light touch massage. The first technique is called the Criss Cross or Figure 8 technique. The Criss Cross technique involves placing the backs of one's fingertips on the opposite sides of the mothers lower back and waist area. The birth partner would then pull their far hand and fingertips towards them, pushing the other way in a criss cross sort of pattern. The technique can be done up the back and then continued back down. One can also use this same idea but move the back of the fingertips in a slow and consistent figure 8 pattern.

The second technique is known as the V's. It involves the same positioning of the partner behind the birth mother using the same fingertip idea starting at the base of the spine. The fingertips of one hand are then placed to make a V and the fingertips of the other hand are slotted inside and moved up towards the top of the neck with slow and consistent motions, repeating as needed over the entire back.

The birth partner needs to explain how the light touch massage technique works so that the mother understands the idea of releasing endorphins. It is up to each individual when and where this kind of technique is used during the birthing process.

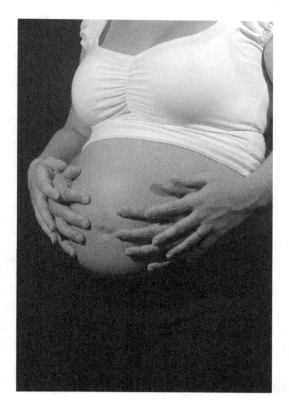

Light Touch Massage Recap

- Using the back of their hand, the birth partner begins at the base of the birth mother's spine drawing a V-shape outwards, moving up to the base of the neck.

- They continue stroking up to the neck, then sweeping down the sides and back up.

- Repeat several times or as desired.

- Can also be done using the palms of the hands creating circles, figure 8's or V's all over the back.

- To complete, the birth partner can then lightly stroke down the spine, starting at the base of the skull down to the tailbone.

Chapter 10 –Meditation Scripts

"The moment a child is born, the mother is also born. She never existed before. The woman existed, but the mother, never. A mother is something absolutely new." – Rajneesh

Lemon Cutting Script

The classic lemon cutting script is a wonderful way to help develop your self-hypnosis skills. This exercise helps one experience a non-birth related state of trance or relaxation.

Each of us processes information differently as we have seen. Some people see things in their mind, some hear things while others enjoy touching things. Try this simple exercise to see which modality you prefer.

The Lemon Cutting Script

Take a deep breath in and close your eyes - continue breathing deeply for 2-3 more breaths - clearing the energy. Allow your breath to travel in through your body, all the way down to your toes then back up. Do this several more times.

Now picture in your mind's eye a beautiful kitchen. This could be a kitchen you are familiar with or one out of your imagination. Practice moving around the kitchen and notice what you see, sense or feel. Touch the counter tops and notice the texture. Look around you and notice anything familiar.

Feel the warmth of the room, and breathe in any aromas. You might notice the smell of coffee brewing or cookies baking. See the steam or condensation forming on the windows. Hear the bubbling sounds of food cooking. Feel the warmth as you open the oven door. Listen for any more sounds or spend some time just observing.

Open the refrigerator and notice what you see, sense or feel. Now go back to the countertop and imagine a beautiful bright yellow lemon sitting on a cutting board. Notice the details, the texture of the skin, the smooth surface and the plumpness. See and feel every one of the pores of this lemon –so smooth - run your fingers over the lemon; notice it's wax like consistency. Study all the features of the lemon.

Imagine that besides the board is a large cutting knife. Give yourself permission to pick up the knife. In your mind's eye see yourself cutting the lemon in half. Watch the juice as it runs down forming small puddles on the board.

Now take half of the lemon and bring it to your nose – smell the aroma.

Now take the lemon and place your teeth into it being aware of the juices. Notice how they run through your mouth. Slowly move your tongue around the inside of your mouth, feel what is happening in your mouth. Be aware of the changes taking place. Smell the lemon, taste the bitterness, and notice what you see, sense or feel.

Open your eyes back up.

Now ask yourself how you processed information as you traveled through the kitchen? Did you notice smells more? Did you notice the texture of the countertop and the feel of the lemon rind more? Maybe you enjoyed simply looking at the scenery and the beautiful colors. Notice which modality you prefer, sight, sound or touch. Ask yourself if you were able to smell the lemon or taste the lemon as well.

Fear Release - Place of Peace Script Exercise

Gently close your eyes... and bring yourself into a very relaxed state. Take in a slow, deep breath - and exhale, breathing down... directing your breath and love downward. Take in another deep breath... exhaling slowly downward again. Now, take in yet another breath... and this time, as you exhale... feel the relaxation spreading through your entire body... especially into your abdomen. As you continue to breathe - feel yourself relaxing deeper... and deeper with each breath.

Now imagine that you are resting somewhere that you really enjoy. You might see yourself lying in a beautiful meadow on a warm and sunny day, on a serene and tranquil beach or floating on a raft on a calm lake, wherever you like. Take yourself somewhere that you feel very safe and relaxed.

Imagine looking up into a clear blue sky – a cloudless blue sky. As you breathe, notice the sights and scents all around you. Feel the air on your cheeks and the sun on your skin. Feel the warmth and the peace and the joy.

You might even feel like you are beginning to drift, and float up into the sky. Enjoy this sensation and freedom of movement. Continue breathing easily and deeply.

Soon all you can see is the blueness surrounding you, the calm sensation filling you as you continue to breathe slowly and deeply. Feel yourself relaxing more and more as you're gradually absorbed, gently absorbed into the blueness and the stillness and the peacefulness.

Now notice how there is a gentle shift from looking into the blue sky to looking into a calm, peaceful, beautiful deep blue sea of color. Far below through the clear, calm blue color you can see a multitude of different shades of blue, and each of these shades of blue becomes deeper and deeper, like the deepest level of relaxation that you can imagine.

Take a moment now and allow yourself to release anything that may be holding you back at this moment in time. Release all the stress, all the worry and all the fear. Just let it all go. You might envision yourself standing under a beautiful waterfall of light. Imagine how soothing this light feels as it eases into your skin and into your pores. Notice how it feels warm and invigorating at the same time.

As you enjoy this shower of light, allow the healing energy to penetrate your soul. Feel the energy as it moves through your body – warming you – and healing you.

Now in this state of peace and joy, begin to visualize a beautiful soft, pink rosebud in the lower portion of your uterus. Imagine your uterus is made up of these beautiful petals. As you begin to relax more and more, notice how this beautiful flower supports your baby – so soft yet so strong. You have so much power and strength. There is nothing you cannot accomplish with faith and love.

Now in this place of healing, notice how good you feel, how radiant you are. Notice how strong and confident you feel about this upcoming event. Release any feelings of doubt you may have at this time. See yourself as confident and amazing. See yourself gently birthing your baby with grace and ease. See yourself easily going through the birthing experience.

Notice all the colors in the scene – notice all the details. See yourself holding your baby with love and joy. Send your baby a silent message – a message of love. See your baby responding with joy. Hold your baby skin to skin – notice how comforting it feels. Hold this photo in your minds eye – and experience the love and the joy.

Now repeat in your mind the following affirmations:

- I trust my body to birth my baby.

- I am relaxed and happy during this process.

- I am focused on a smooth and calm birth.

- I welcome my baby with love.

Just enjoy the beauty and the peace and the calm that you now feel. Sit for a moment and let your consciousness drift.

Thank your mind and body for cooperating today and participating in this beautiful journey. Send your baby love and kindness and compassion. Celebrate this moment.

And when you are ready, take one more long slow deep breath and become aware of the sounds around you.

Now gently open your eyes and come back to where you are - knowing that you have now released all of your fears and concerns.

Special Fear Release Audio Meditation

I have prepared for you special *Fear Release* recording, the best of my HypnoBirthing AudioScripts© that I all created myself with lots of love. I am sure you will find it useful. Please use it best if lying or sitting comfortably. You should use stereo headphones as specific messages are designed to go to specific hemispheres of your brain and without stereo headphones you will likely not get the best results. Laying down is best but a sitting on the confortable chair or sitting place is OK as long as you have head support and your eyes are closed.

Please do not perform any type of activity while listening, often your mind will try to cheat you saying 'I could do something useful around the house, iron and listen in the same time, it is just fine..." or 'I hear this nicely also when I prepare a dinner..." etc. Do not fall to these tricks because, laying down with your eyes closed and using stereo headphones at a comfortable volume is the best and most effective way to listen and prepare your conscious and subconscious mind. Last and strongest warning - **Do not drive or operate with anything potentially dangerous while listening**.

I will certainly appreciate your comments and experiences (about the audio and the book as well) feel free to share both as a review of this book. From experience I can tell that your words will mean a lot to other women that are maybe not enough strong or decisive. Thank You!

Instructions for Downloading Fear release Audio Meditation

I tried to make this even simpler however due to anti spam laws, regulations and what not, there are few steps that most of you are probably familiar with.

1) Type in this Link http://eepurl.com/Ome5T in to your browser.

2) Opt in the form your email and fist name there, and be sure I will not spam you, or misuse your information in any way, nor I'll allow anyone else to do so.

3) I will send you (well automated service I had to purchase) will send you immediately email where you have to confirm your subscription.

4) When you do, please allow up to one hour and you will receive email from me with the download link. There will be no preview option, only download and that is what you need.

Word of Warning: The file will have a weird name, something long and without any meaning, something just as 'w5df5wsgjbasdfgh332da.mp3' for example. This is done with purpose, in order to prevent unauthorized downloads. Once you download it on you computer or device, best is you rename the file so that you can find it without the problem whenever you want to start listening the meditation.

Chapter 11 – Is HypnoBirthing Right for You?

"The major role that the body's natural oxytocin plays in birth encourages the idea that birth is an experience of love... Birth is a spiritual experience simply because it is largely an act of love on the part of the body physiology and the indwelling spirit." - Cathy Daub

I hope this brief introduction into the process of HypnoBirthing has been helpful. Knowledge is power and you are now armed with all of the most important facts.

HypnoBirthing is an option and a choice. Whether you choose to exercise this option is up to you. If you have a desire to birth your baby naturally and calmly, then HypnoBirthing may be a good choice for you.

HypnoBirthing is a natural and effective way to birth your baby because it gives you some very powerful tools that you can use during the labor and delivery process. HypnoBirthing uses hypnosis, i.e. the power of the mind, to help you enter into and stay in a very relaxed and calm state of mind. The more calm and relaxed you are, the better your birth experience will be.

HypnoBirthing helps you tap into your natural healing abilities and it is a wonderful pain management tool as well. HypnoBirthing helps you do what you are naturally designed to do – birth your baby in a natural and comfortable way.

The process you have learned has merely skimmed the surface of what HypnoBirthing is all about. Through education and awareness you become more aware of your options. **The techniques learned in HypnoBirthing can help you in many areas of life, because they help you tap into your body's natural healing abilities.** When there is fear about birth or fear when it comes to parenting, the body tends to reflect this fear by tensing up – triggering the fight or flight response. This in turn leads to tight and constricted muscles. Arming yourself with the knowledge and power that HypnoBirthing offers allows you to eliminate those fears and concerns.

HypnoBirthing aims to educate both the birth mother and the birth partner about what causes pain – and it teaches you that birth doesn't have to be a painful and dreaded experience. Using the techniques given like self-hypnosis and deep breathing, you can become much more aware of what your body is capable of.

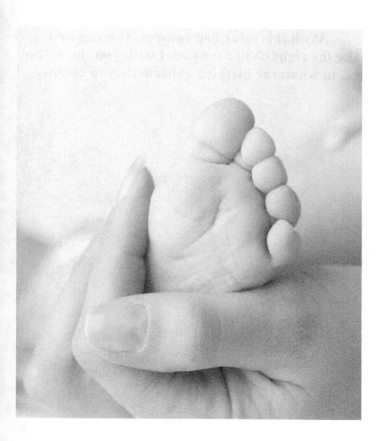

From empowering yourself through the proper use of language to practicing visual, auditory and kinesthetic techniques, HypnoBirthing allows you to take back control. It allows you to be truly involved in your baby's birth, as opposed to letting the fear of the unknown take over.

With this informed consent, you can now make the right choice for you. I wish you the best of luck, in whatever birthing experience you choose.

Made in United States
Orlando, FL
28 October 2023